RHEUMATOID

ARTHRITIS DIET

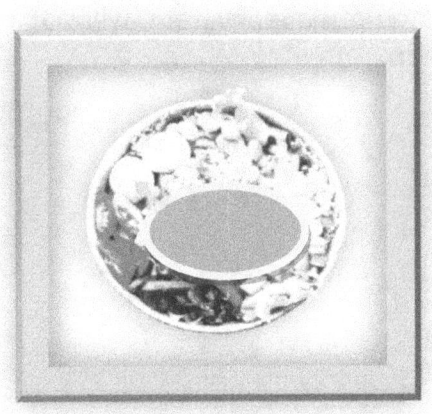

Nutrition Guide and 100 Anti-Inflammatory
Recipes to Fight Flares, Fatigue And Manage
Symptom

Nancy J. Atkins.

Copyright

INTRODUCTION

Do the gnawing aches in your joints whisper secrets of frustration and fatigue? Does the morning stiffness make even simple tasks feel like scaling a mountain? You're not alone. Millions worldwide share the daily struggle of arthritis, a relentless foe that steals joy and mobility.

Believe me, I understand. The pain, the exhaustion, the feeling of being trapped in your own body—I've seen it firsthand. Not just in patients, but in the woman I love most: my mother. Watching her battle with arthritis, her spirit dimming with each flare-up, was a fire that fueled my passion to find answers.

But here's the truth: Arthritis doesn't have to rule your life. As a qualified dietitian with over 15 years of experience, I've witnessed the transformative power of food. It wasn't a magic cure, but for my mother and countless others, it was a game-changer. Through simple dietary adjustments, we unlocked a path to reduced inflammation, increased energy, and a renewed zest for life.

This book isn't just a collection of recipes; it's a beacon of hope and a roadmap to reclaiming your well-being. It's the story of my mother, your story, and the countless others who have found relief through the power of my diet. It's a journey towards a lifeless life defined by pain and more filled with possibility.

Are you ready to take that first step? Let's embark on this adventure together. Open this book and discover the delicious secrets that I used to heal my mother and every one of my patients. Remember, you are not alone. And together, we can rewrite the narrative of your journey with arthritis.

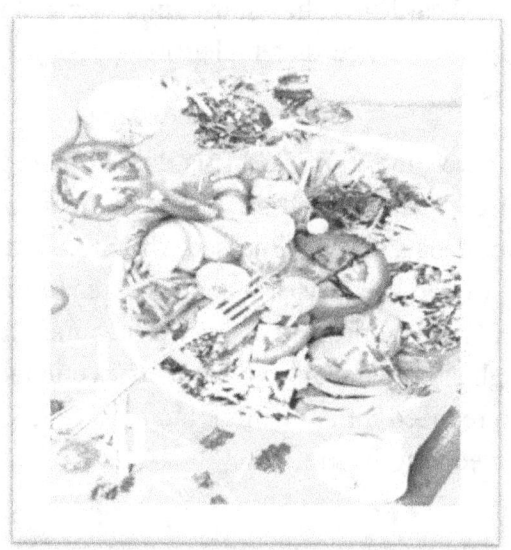

CHAPTER 1

Understanding Rheumatoid Arthritis and Diet Management

What is rheumatoid arthritis?

Rheumatoid arthritis (RA) is an inflammatory illness that causes chronic inflammation in the joints. Unlike osteoarthritis, which is caused by wear and tear, RA affects the synovial lining of the joints, resulting in swelling, discomfort, stiffness, and eventual joint destruction. While the specific etiology is unknown, genetic and environmental factors are thought to contribute to its development.

The Role of Diet in Rheumatoid Arthritis

While there is no treatment for RA, controlling symptoms and delaying disease progression are critical. The diet plays an important role in this process. Certain foods have inflammatory qualities that can exacerbate symptoms, whereas others have anti-inflammatory properties that can reduce pain and stiffness. A well-balanced diet rich in key nutrients can help people with RA maintain their overall health and well-being.

Causes and symptoms:

The exact cause of RA is unknown, but it is thought to entail both genetics and environmental factors. Common symptoms include joint discomfort, edema, stiffness, and warmth, which can affect hands, feet, and wrists symmetrically.

Common symptoms include fatigue, low-grade fever, loss of appetite, and weight loss. Severe instances may also cause lung or eye difficulties.

Impact in Daily Life:

RA can have a major influence on daily activities because of pain, stiffness, and fatigue. It can have an impact on one's career, relationships, and overall well-being.

The role of inflammation in rheumatoid arthritis:

Chronic inflammation is a characteristic of RA. The immune system incorrectly assaults the synovium, causing inflammation, tissue damage, and discomfort. Certain dietary choices can impact inflammatory pathways, perhaps resulting in advantages.

Relationship between Diet and Rheumatoid Arthritis

Inflammatory Foods:

Foods high in saturated and Trans fats, processed carbs, and added sweets can increase inflammation and exacerbate RA symptoms. These include processed meats, sugary beverages, fried foods, and pastries.

Anti-inflammatory Foods

Foods high in omega-3 fatty acids, antioxidants, and fiber have anti-inflammatory benefits. This includes:

Fatty fish: salmon, tuna, and mackerel.

Foods and vegetables: berries, leafy greens, and vitamin C-rich foods.

Nuts and seeds include almonds, walnuts, and flaxseeds.

The whole grains include brown rice, quinoa, and oats.

How Diet Influences Joint Health:

Anti-inflammatory foods can alleviate pain and stiffness, improve joint mobility, and boost overall health and energy levels.

Important of Nutrients for Managing Rheumatoid Arthritis

Omega-3 Fatty Acids:

Omega-3s, found in fatty fish, have powerful anti-inflammatory qualities and may help relieve morning stiffness and joint pain.

Vitamins and Minerals:

Vitamins C, D, and E, as well as the minerals zinc and selenium, work as antioxidants, reducing inflammation and promoting immunological function.

Importance of a Balanced Diet: A balanced diet provides important nutrients while minimizing inflammatory triggers.

Foods to Eat For Arthritis

Fat Fish:

Aim for 2-3 servings each week to reap omega-3 advantages.

Berries: High in antioxidants and fiber, they have anti-inflammatory properties.

leafy greens.

They promote general health by being high in vitamins, minerals, and fiber.

Nuts and Seeds: Contain healthful fats, fiber, and nutrients.

Whole Grains: High in fiber and complex carbs, they provide lasting energy.

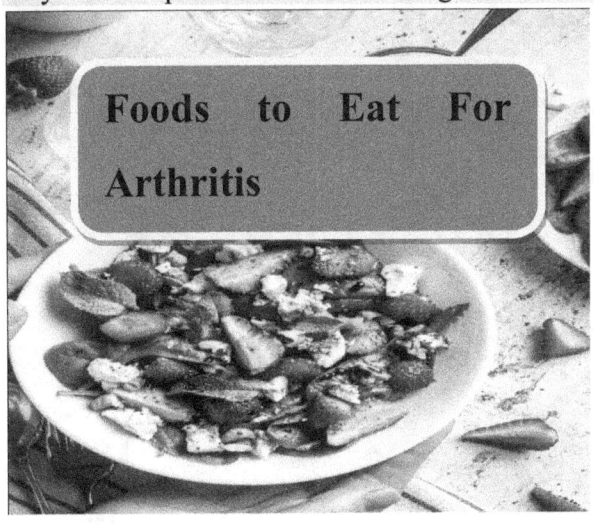

Foods to Eat For Arthritis

Foods To You Need To Avoid.

Processed food:

High in saturated and Trans fats, salt, and added sugars, these foods lead to inflammation.6.2 Red Meat: Reduce your intake of rd meat as it may have pro-inflammatory effects.

Sugary Drinks: Sugary drinks cause inflammation and weight gain, increasing RA symptoms.

Remember, dietary modifications alone cannot cure RA; however, including anti-inflammatory foods and reducing inflammatory triggers can be a useful element of managing the disease.

CHAPTER 2

Delicious Breakfast Recipes for Arthritis

Berries and Yogurt Parfait

Preparation Time: 5 minutes

Ingredients:

- 1/2 cup plain Greek yogurt

- 1/2 cup mixed berries (fresh or frozen)

- 1/4 cup granola

- 1 tablespoon chia seeds (optional)

- Honey or maple syrup (optional, to taste)

Instructions:

1. Layer yogurt, berries, and granola in a glass or jar.

2. Sprinkle with chia seeds, if desired.

3. Drizzle with honey or maple syrup for added sweetness (optional).

Nutritional Value: (per serving)

- Calories: 250-300

- Protein: 10-15g

- Fiber: 5-10g

- Fat: 5–10g (depending on yogurt and toppings)

- Antioxidants: from berries and chia seeds

- Calcium: from yogurt

Turmeric Oatmeal with Nuts and Seeds

Preparation Time: 15 minutes

Ingredients:

- 1/2 cup rolled oats

- 1 cup of water or milk

- 1/4 teaspoon turmeric powder

- Pinch of black pepper

- Use 1/4 cup of chopped nuts (walnuts, almonds, pecans).

- 1 tablespoon seeds (chia, flax, sunflower)

- Fresh fruit (optional)

Instructions:

1. Bring water or milk to a boil in a saucepan.

2. Add oats, turmeric, and black pepper. Stir occasionally after you have reduced the heat and simmered for 5 minutes.

3. Remove from heat and stir in nuts and seeds.

4. Top with fresh fruit, if desired.

Nutritional Value: (per serving)

- Calories: 300-350

- Protein: 5-10g

- Fiber: 8-10g

- Fat: 10–15g (depending on nuts and seeds)

- Antioxidants: from turmeric and fruits (optional)

- Iron: from oats

Smoked Salmon Scramble with Avocado:

Preparation Time: 10 minutes

Ingredients:

- 2 eggs

- 1 tablespoon of milk

- 1/4 cup smoked salmon, flaked

- 1/4 avocado, mashed

- Salt and pepper to taste

- Optional toppings: chopped chives, dill, and hot sauce

Instructions:

1. Whisk the eggs and milk in a bowl.

2. Heat a pan with oil or butter over medium heat.

3. Pour in the egg mixture and scramble until cooked through.

4. Add the smoked salmon and cook for another minute.

5. Remove from heat and stir in avocado.

6. You have to season with salt and pepper to get a good taste.

7. Top with chives, dill, or hot sauce, if desired.

Nutritional Value: (per serving)

- Calories: 300-350

- Protein: 20-25g

- Fat: 20–25g (depending on oil and avocado)

- Omega-3s: From smoked salmon

- Vitamins A, C, and E: from avocado

Green Smoothie with Protein Powder:

Preparation Time: 5 minutes

Ingredients:

- Use 1 cup of leafy greens (spinach, kale, and romaine).

- 1/2 cup banana, frozen or fresh

- 1/2 cup of water or milk

- 1 scoop of protein powder (optional)

- 1 tablespoon nut butter (optional)

- Honey or maple syrup (optional, to taste)

Instructions:

1. Make sure to blend all ingredients in a blender until they are smooth.

2. Add more water or milk if needed for the desired consistency.

3. Adjust sweetness with honey or maple syrup if desired.

Nutritional Value: (per serving)

- Calories: 200–300 (depending on ingredients)

- Protein: 15-20g (with protein powder)

- Fiber: 5-10g

- Vitamins A, C, and K: From leafy greens

- Potassium: from bananas

Cottage Cheese Toast with Cucumber and Tomato:

Preparation Time: 5 minutes

Ingredients:

- 1 slice of whole-wheat toast

- 1/4 cup cottage cheese

- 1/4 cucumber, sliced

- 1/4 tomato, sliced

- Salt and pepper to taste

- Optional toppings: fresh herbs, avocado slices

Instructions:

1. Toast bread.

2. Spread cottage cheese on toast.

3. Top with cucumber and tomato slices.

4. You have to season with salt and pepper to get a good taste.

5. Add optional toppings if desired.

Nutritional Value: (per serving)

- Calories: 2

Veggie Breakfast Burrito:

Preparation Time: 15 minutes

Ingredients:

- 1 whole-wheat tortilla

- 1/2 cup scrambled eggs

- 1/4 cup black beans, mashed or rinsed and drained

- Use 1/4 cup of chopped vegetables (bell peppers, onions, mushrooms, and spinach).

- 1/4 avocado, sliced

- 1 tablespoon salsa (optional)

- Salt and pepper to taste

Instructions:

1. Warm a tortilla in a pan or microwave.

2. Spread scrambled eggs onto the tortilla.

3. Top with black beans, vegetables, avocado, and salsa (optional).

4. You have to season with salt and pepper to get a good taste.

5. Roll up the tortilla and enjoy.

Nutritional Value: (per serving)

- Calories: 300-350

- Protein: 15-20g

- Fiber: 5-10g

- Fat: 10–15g (depending on avocado)

- Antioxidants: from vegetables

Green Smoothie Bowl:

Preparation Time: 5 minutes

Ingredients:

- Use 1 cup of leafy greens (spinach, kale, and romaine).

- 1/2 cup frozen banana

- 1/2 cup of water or milk

- 1 tablespoon nut butter (optional)

- 1/4 cup granola

- Fresh fruit (berries, mango, pineapple)

- Chia seeds (optional)

Instructions:

1. Blend leafy greens, bananas, water or milk, and nut butter (optional) in a blender until smooth.

2. Pour the smoothie into a bowl.

3. Top with granola, fresh fruit, and chia seeds (optional).

Nutritional Value: (per serving)

- Calories: 250–300 (depending on ingredients)

- Protein: 5–10g (with nut butter)

- Fiber: 5-10g

- Vitamins A, C, and K: From leafy greens

- Potassium: from bananas

Rice Pudding with Almonds:

Preparation Time: 30 minutes

Ingredients:

- 1/2 cup brown rice, cooked

- 1 cup of milk

- 1/4 cup of water

- 1/4 cup raisins

- 1 tablespoon of honey or maple syrup

- 1/4 teaspoon cinnamon

- 1/4 cup sliced almonds

Instructions:

1. Combine cooked rice, milk, water, raisins, honey, and cinnamon in a saucepan.

2. Bring to a boil, then reduce heat and simmer for 20 minutes, stirring occasionally, until the rice is creamy and most of the liquid is absorbed.

3. Remove from heat and stir in almonds.

4. Serve it warm or chilled.

Nutritional Value: (per serving)

- Calories: 300-350

- Protein: 5-10g

- Fiber: 5-10g

- Calcium: from milk

- Iron: from brown rice

Spinach and Feta Pancake:

Preparation Time: 15 minutes

Ingredients:

- 1 cup all-purpose flour

- 1 teaspoon baking powder

- 1/4 teaspoon salt

- 1 cup of milk

- 1 egg

- 1/2 cup chopped spinach

- 1/4 cup crumbled feta cheese

- Olive oil for cooking

Instructions:

1. In a bowl Whisk flour, baking powder, and salt together.

2. In a separate bowl, whisk together the milk, egg, and spinach.

3. Fold the wet ingredients into the dry ingredients until just combined.

4. Stir in feta cheese.

5. Heat olive oil in a pan over medium heat.

6. Pour the batter onto the pan and cook for 2-3 minutes per side, or until golden brown and cooked through.

7. Serve immediately.

Nutritional Value: (per serving)

- Calories: 300-350

- Protein: 15-20g

- Fiber: 5-10g

- Calcium: from feta cheese

- Iron: from spinach

Breakfast Quinoa Stuffed Bell Pepper:

Preparation Time: 45 minutes

Ingredients:

- 1 bell pepper, halved and seeds removed

- 1/2 cup cooked quinoa

- 1/4 cup black beans, mashed or rinsed and drained

- 1/4 cup chopped vegetables (corn, peppers, onions)

- 1/4 cup cottage cheese

- 1 tablespoon chopped herbs (cilantro, parsley)

- Salt and pepper to taste

Instructions:

1. Preheat the oven to 375°F (190°C).

2. Place halved bell peppers, cut side down, on a baking sheet. Bake for 10–15 minutes, or until slightly softened.

3. Meanwhile, combine cooked quinoa, black beans, chopped vegetables, cottage cheese, and herbs in a bowl. Season with salt and pepper, to taste.

4. Remove the softened bell peppers from the oven and fill each half with the quinoa mixture.

5. Bake for an additional 20–25 minutes, or until bell peppers are tender and filling is heated through.

6. Serve immediately, garnished with additional herbs or hot sauce (optional).

Nutritional Value (per serving):

- Calories: 300-350

- Protein: 15-20g

- Fiber: 5-10g

- Fat: 5–10g (depending on cheese)

- Vitamins and minerals: from vegetables and bell peppers

Chia Seed Pudding with Fruit and Nuts:

Preparation Time: 10 minutes (plus overnight soaking)

Ingredients:

- 1/4 cup chia seeds

- 1 cup milk (dairy or plant-based)

- 1/4 teaspoon vanilla extract (optional)

- 1/4 cup chopped nuts (almonds, walnuts, pecans)

- 1/4 cup fresh fruit (berries, mango, or pineapple)

- Use 1 tablespoon of honey or maple syrup (optional).

Instructions:

1. In a jar or container, combine chia seeds, milk, and vanilla extract (optional). Stir well and refrigerate overnight.

2. In the morning, stir in chopped nuts and fresh fruit.

3. Drizzle with honey or maple syrup for added sweetness (optional).

Nutritional Value: (per serving)

- Calories: 250-300

- Protein: 5-10g

- Fiber: 10-15g

- Fat: 10–15g (depending on nuts)

- Antioxidants: From fruit

- Calcium: from milk

Whole-Wheat Pancakes with Yogurt and Berries:

Preparation Time: 20 minutes

Ingredients:

- 1 cup whole-wheat flour

- 1 teaspoon baking powder

- 1/2 teaspoon salt

- 1 cup milk (dairy or plant-based)

- 1 egg

- 1 tablespoon of olive oil

- 1/2 cup plain yogurt

- 1/4 cup fresh berries

Instructions:

1. In a bowl, whisk together flour, baking powder, and salt.

2. In a separate bowl, whisk together the milk, egg, and olive oil.

3. Combine the wet ingredients with the dry ingredients, mixing until just combined.

4. Over medium heat, you have to Heat a lightly greased pan. Pour the batter onto the pan, forming small pancakes.

5. Cook for 2-3 minutes per side, or until golden brown and cooked through.

6. Serve pancakes topped with yogurt and fresh berries.

Nutritional Value: (per serving)

- Calories: 300-350

- Protein: 15-20g

- Fiber: 5-10g

- Fat: 10–15g (depending on cooking oil)

- Calcium: from yogurt

- Vitamins: from berries

Scrambled Tofu with Vegetables:

Preparation Time: 15 minutes

Ingredients:

- 1 block (14 oz) of firm tofu, drained and crumbled

- 1/2 teaspoon turmeric powder

- 1/4 teaspoon black pepper

- 1 tablespoon of olive oil

- Use 1/2 cup of chopped vegetables (bell peppers, onions, mushrooms).

- 1/4 cup spinach, chopped

- Salt and pepper to taste

Instructions:

1. In a bowl, crumble the tofu and toss with turmeric and black pepper.

2. Over medium heat, you need to heat olive oil in a pan.

3. Add crumbled tofu and cook for 5-7 minutes, stirring occasionally, until golden brown.

4. Add the chopped vegetables and cook for another 5 minutes, or until softened.

5. Stir in the spinach and cook until wilted.

6. You need to season with salt and pepper to get a good taste.

7. Serve immediately.

Nutritional Value: (per serving)

- Calories: 250-300

- Protein: 20-25g

- Fiber: 5-10g

- Fat: 10–15g (depending on olive oil)

- Antioxidants: from turmeric and vegetables

Mediterranean Omelet:

Preparation Time: 20 minutes

Ingredients:

- 2 eggs

- 1 tablespoon of olive oil

- 1/4 cup chopped spinach

- 1/4 cup crumbled feta cheese

- 1/4 cup chopped sundried tomatoes

- Salt and pepper to taste

- Optional toppings: fresh herbs (dill, parsley)

Instructions:

1. Whisk eggs in a bowl.

2. Over medium heat, you need to heat olive oil in a pan.

3. Pour the egg mixture into the pan and swirl to coat the bottom.

4. Spread spinach over the eggs.

5. Sprinkle with feta cheese and sundried tomatoes.

6. Cook for 3-5 minutes, or until eggs are almost set.

7. You need to fold the omelet in half and cook it for another minute.

8. Then season with salt and pepper to get a good taste.

9. Top with optional fresh herbs before serving.

Nutritional Value: (per serving)

- Calories: 300-350

- Protein: 20-25g

Tropical Yogurt Bowl:

Preparation Time: 5 minutes

Ingredients:

- Use 1/2 cup of plain yogurt (dairy or plant-based).

- 1/2 cup diced mango

- 1/2 cup diced pineapple

- 1/2 cup diced papaya

- 1/4 cup granola

- 1 tablespoon chia seeds (optional)

- Honey or maple syrup (optional, to taste)

Instructions:

1. In a bowl, combine yogurt, diced fruits, and granola.

2. Sprinkle with chia seeds, if desired.

3. Drizzle with honey or maple syrup for added sweetness (optional).

Nutritional Value: (per serving)

- Calories: 300-350

- Protein: 10-15g

- Fiber: 5-10g

- Fat: 5–10g (depending on yogurt)

- Vitamins C and A: From fruits

Quinoa Power Bowl:

Preparation Time: 20 minutes (plus cooking quinoa)

Ingredients:

- 1 cup of cooked quinoa

- 1/2 cup roasted vegetables (sweet potatoes, broccoli, chickpeas)

- 1/4 cup chopped avocado

- 1/4 cup chopped fresh herbs (cilantro, parsley)

- 1 tablespoon of olive oil

- 1 tablespoon of lemon juice

- Salt and pepper to taste

Instructions:

1. Prepare quinoa according to package instructions.

2. Roast vegetables (if not already prepared) at 400°F for 20–25 minutes, until tender.

3. In a bowl, combine quinoa, roasted vegetables, avocado, and herbs.

4. Drizzle with olive oil and lemon juice.

5. Season with salt and pepper, to taste.

Nutritional Value: (per serving)

- Calories: 350-400

- Protein: 15-20g

- Fiber: 8-10g

CHAPTER 3

Loaded Nutritious Lunch Recipes
Black Bean-Quinoa Bowl

Preparation Time: 15 minutes

Ingredients:

- 1 cup quinoa, rinsed
- 2 cups cooked black beans
- Use 1 cup of corn kernels (fresh or frozen).
- 1 cup cherry tomatoes, halved
- 1 avocado, diced
- 1/4 cup red onion, finely chopped
- 1/4 cup cilantro, chopped
- Juice of 1 lime
- Salt and pepper to taste

Instructions:

1. Cook quinoa according to package instructions.

2. In a large bowl, combine cooked quinoa, black beans, corn, cherry tomatoes, avocado, red onion, and cilantro.

3. Squeeze lime juice over the mixture and toss gently to combine.

4. You need to season with salt and pepper to get a good taste.

5. Serve immediately or refrigerate for later.

Nutritional Value (per serving):

- Calories: 400

- Protein: 15g

- Carbohydrates: 65g

- Fat: 10g

- Fiber: 12g

Veggie & Hummus Sandwich

Preparation Time:

- 10 minutes

Ingredients:

- 4 slices of whole-grain bread

- 1/2 cup hummus

- 1 cucumber, thinly sliced

- 1 large tomato, sliced

- 1 cup of spinach leaves

- Use 1/4 cup red bell pepper, thinly sliced.
- Salt and pepper to taste

Instructions:

1. Spread hummus evenly on each slice of bread.
2. Layer cucumber, tomato, spinach, and red bell pepper on two slices of bread.
3. Season with salt and pepper.
4. Top with the remaining slices of bread to make two sandwiches.
5. Cut in half and serve.

Nutritional Value (per sandwich):

- Calories: 350
- Protein: 12g
- Carbohydrates: 45g
- Fat: 15g
- Fiber: 8g

Lemony Lentil Salad with Feta

Preparation Time:

- 20 minutes

Ingredients:

- 1 cup dried green lentils, cooked and cooled
- 1/2 cup feta cheese, crumbled
- 1 cucumber, diced
- 1 cup cherry tomatoes, halved
- 1/4 cup red onion, finely chopped
- 2 tablespoons fresh parsley, chopped
- Zest and juice of 1 lemon
- 3 tablespoons of olive oil
- Salt and pepper to taste

Instructions:

1. In a large bowl, combine lentils, feta, cucumber, cherry tomatoes, red onion, and parsley.
2. In a small bowl, whisk together lemon zest, lemon juice, olive oil, salt, and pepper.
3. Pour the dressing over the lentil mixture and toss gently to coat.
4. Serve chilled.

Nutritional Value (per serving):

- Calories: 320

- Protein: 15g
- Carbohydrates: 35g
- Fat: 15g
- Fiber: 12g

Chickpea Tuna Salad

Preparation Time:

- 15 minutes

Ingredients:

- 2 cans chickpeas, drained and rinsed
- 1/4 cup mayonnaise
- 2 tablespoons Dijon mustard
- 1 celery stalk, finely chopped
- 1/4 cup red onion, finely chopped
- 2 tablespoons fresh dill, chopped
- Salt and pepper to taste

Instructions:

1. In a large bowl, mash chickpeas with a fork or potato masher.
2. Add mayonnaise, Dijon mustard, celery, red onion, and dill. Mix well.

3. You need to season with salt and pepper to get a good taste.

4. Refrigerate for at least 30 minutes before serving.

5. Serve on bread, crackers, or as a salad.

Nutritional Value (per serving):

- Calories: 280
- Protein: 10g
- Carbohydrates: 30g
- Fat: 15g
- Fiber: 8g

Cucumber and Avocado Sandwich

Preparation Time:

- 12 minutes

Ingredients:

- 4 slices of whole-grain bread
- 1 large cucumber, thinly sliced
- 1 avocado, sliced
- 1/4 cup hummus
- 1/4 cup feta cheese, crumbled

- 1/4 cup sun-dried tomatoes, chopped

- 2 tablespoons of pumpkin seeds

- Salt and pepper to taste

Instructions:

1. Spread hummus evenly on each slice of bread.

2. Layer cucumber, avocado, feta, sun-dried tomatoes, and pumpkin seeds on two slices of bread.

3. Season with salt and pepper.

4. Top with the remaining slices of bread to make two sandwiches.

5. Cut in half and serve.

Nutritional Value (per sandwich):

- Calories: 380

- Protein: 12g

- Carbohydrates: 45g

- Fat: 18g

- Fiber: 10g

Avocado Tuna Spinach Salad:

Preparation Time:

- 15 minutes

Ingredients:

- 1 can (5 oz) tuna, drained
- 2 avocados, diced
- 2 cups of fresh spinach
- 1 cup cherry tomatoes, halved
- 1/4 cup red onion, thinly sliced
- 2 tablespoons of olive oil
- 1 tablespoon of lemon juice
- Salt and pepper to taste

Instructions:

1. In a large bowl, combine tuna, diced avocados, fresh spinach, cherry tomatoes, and red onion.
2. You need to whisk together, in a small bowl, olive oil, lemon juice, salt, and pepper.
3. To combine, you need to Pour the dressing over the salad and toss gently.
4. Serve immediately, and enjoy!

Nutritional Value:

Calories: 350

- Protein: 20g
- Fat: 25g
- Carbohydrates: 15g
- Fiber: 8g

Vegan Burrito Bowls with Cauliflower Rice:

Preparation Time:

- 30 minutes

Ingredients:

- 2 cups of cauliflower rice
- Use 1 can of black beans, drain it, and rinse it.
- 1 cup of corn kernels
- 1 cup cherry tomatoes, quartered
- 1 avocado, sliced
- 1/2 cup red onion, finely chopped
- 1/4 cup fresh cilantro, chopped
- 1 lime, juiced
- 1 teaspoon of cumin

- Salt and pepper to taste

Instructions:

1. In a skillet, sauté cauliflower rice with cumin, salt, and pepper until tender.
2. Assemble bowls with cauliflower rice, black beans, corn, cherry tomatoes, avocado slices, and red onion.
3. Drizzle lime juice over the bowls and sprinkle with fresh cilantro.
4. Serve and enjoy your vegan burrito bowls!

Nutritional Value

Calories: 400

- Protein: 15g
- Fat: 10g
- Carbohydrates: 65g
- Fiber: 18g

White Bean and Veggie Salad:

Preparation Time:

- 20 minutes

Ingredients:

- Use 1 can of (15 oz) white beans, drained and rinsed.

- 1 cucumber, diced

- 1 bell pepper, diced

- 1 cup cherry tomatoes, halved

- 1/2 red onion, finely chopped

- 1/4 cup feta cheese, crumbled

- 2 tablespoons of olive oil

- 1 tablespoon balsamic vinegar

- Fresh basil leaves for garnish

- Salt and pepper to taste

Instructions:

1. In a large bowl, combine white beans, cucumber, bell pepper, cherry tomatoes, red onion, and feta cheese.

2. You need to whisk together, in a small bowl, olive oil, balsamic vinegar, salt, and pepper.

3. To combine, you need to Pour the dressing over the salad and toss gently.

4. Garnish with fresh basil leaves, and serve.

Nutritional Value

Calories: 300

- Protein: 12g
- Fat: 10g
- Carbohydrates: 45g
- Fiber: 12g

Mediterranean Tuna-Spinach Salad:

Preparation Time:

- 25 minutes

Ingredients:

- 1 can (5 oz) tuna, drained
- 2 cups of fresh spinach
- 1 cup cherry tomatoes, halved
- 1/2 cucumber, sliced
- Use 1/4 cup of Kalamata olives, pitted and sliced.
- 1/4 cup feta cheese, crumbled
- 2 tablespoons of olive oil
- 1 tablespoon of red wine vinegar
- 1 teaspoon dried oregano
- Salt and pepper to taste

Instructions:

1. In a large bowl, combine tuna, fresh spinach, cherry tomatoes, cucumber, Kalamata olives, and feta cheese.

2. You need to whisk together, in a small bowl, olive oil, red wine vinegar, dried oregano, salt, and pepper.

3. To combine, you need to pour the dressing over the salad and toss gently.

4. Serve and enjoy the Mediterranean flavors!

Nutritional Value: Calories: 320

- Protein: 18g
- Fat: 20g
- Carbohydrates: 15g
- Fiber: 5g

White Bean and Avocado Sandwich:

Preparation Time:

- 15 minutes

Ingredients:

- 1 can (15 oz) white beans, drained and mashed

- 1 avocado, mashed
- 1/4 cup red onion, finely chopped
- 1/4 cup fresh cilantro, chopped
- 1 tablespoon of lime juice
- Salt and pepper to taste
- Bread slices (of your choice)
- Lettuce leaves, tomato slices, and any desired toppings

Instructions:

1. In a bowl, combine mashed white beans, mashed avocado, red onion, cilantro, lime juice, salt, and pepper.
2. Spread the mixture onto bread slices.
3. Top with lettuce leaves, tomato slices, and any desired toppings.
4. Assemble the sandwiches and serve.

Nutritional Value: Calories: 300

- Protein: 12g
- Fat: 10g
- Carbohydrates: 45g
- Fiber: 12g

Turkey Cobb Salad:

Preparation Time:

- 20 minutes

Ingredients:

- 2 cups mixed salad greens
- 1 cup cooked turkey breast, diced
- 1 avocado, sliced
- 1 cup cherry tomatoes, halved
- 1/2 cup blue cheese, crumbled
- 2 hard-boiled eggs, sliced
- 1/4 cup bacon bits
- Your favorite salad dressing

Instructions:

1. Arrange salad greens on a plate or in a bowl.

2. Top with diced turkey, avocado slices, cherry tomatoes, blue cheese, sliced hard-boiled eggs, and bacon bits.

3. Drizzle with your favorite salad dressing.

4. Toss gently and serve.

Nutritional Value Calories: 450

- Protein: 30g
- Fat: 25g
- Carbohydrates: 20g
- Fiber: 6g

Thai-Style Chopped Salad with Sriracha Tofu:

Preparation Time:

- 30 minutes

Ingredients:

- 1 block of tofu, pressed and cubed
- 2 tablespoons of soy sauce
- 1 tablespoon Sriracha sauce
- 4 cups of mixed salad greens
- 1 cup of shredded cabbage
- 1 carrot, julienned
- 1 cucumber, sliced
- 1/4 cup fresh cilantro, chopped
- 1/4 cup peanuts, chopped

- Thai peanut dressing

Instructions:

1. Toss tofu cubes with soy sauce and Sriracha, then bake or pan-fry until crispy.

2. In a large bowl, combine salad greens, shredded cabbage, julienned carrot, sliced cucumber, and chopped cilantro.

3. Top with crispy tofu and chopped peanuts.

4. Drizzle with Thai peanut dressing, toss gently, and serve.

Nutritional Value: Calories: 380

- Protein: 20g
- Fat: 20g
- Carbohydrates: 30g
- Fiber: 8g

Chickpea Sunflower Sandwich:

Preparation Time:

- 15 minutes

Ingredients:

- 1 can (15 oz) chickpeas, drained and mashed
- 1/4 cup sunflower seeds
- 2 tablespoons vegan mayo
- 1 tablespoon Dijon mustard
- 1 celery stalk, finely chopped
- 1 green onion, sliced
- Salt and pepper to taste
- Bread slices (of your choice)
- Lettuce leaves, tomato slices, and any desired toppings

Instructions:

1. In a bowl, combine mashed chickpeas, sunflower seeds, vegan mayo, Dijon mustard, celery, green onion, salt, and pepper.
2. Spread the mixture onto bread slices.
3. Top with lettuce leaves, tomato slices, and any desired toppings.
4. Assemble the sandwiches and serve.

Nutritional Value:

Calories: 320

- Protein: 15g
- Fat: 15g
- Carbohydrates: 40g
- Fiber: 10g

Strawberry Avocado Grilled Chicken Salad:

Preparation Time:

- 25 minutes

Ingredients:

- 2 boneless, skinless chicken breasts
- 1 tablespoon of olive oil
- Salt and pepper to taste
- 4 cups of mixed salad greens
- 1 cup strawberries, sliced
- 1 avocado, sliced
- 1/4 cup feta cheese, crumbled
- 1/4 cup balsamic vinaigrette dressing

Instructions:

1. Season chicken breasts with olive oil, salt, and pepper. Grill until fully cooked.

2. Slice the grilled chicken into strips.

3. In a large bowl, combine salad greens, sliced strawberries, sliced avocado, and crumbled feta cheese.

4. Top with grilled chicken strips and drizzle with balsamic vinaigrette dressing.

5. Toss gently and serve.

Nutritional Value: Calories: 400

- Protein: 25g
- Fat: 20g
- Carbohydrates: 30g
- Fiber: 8g

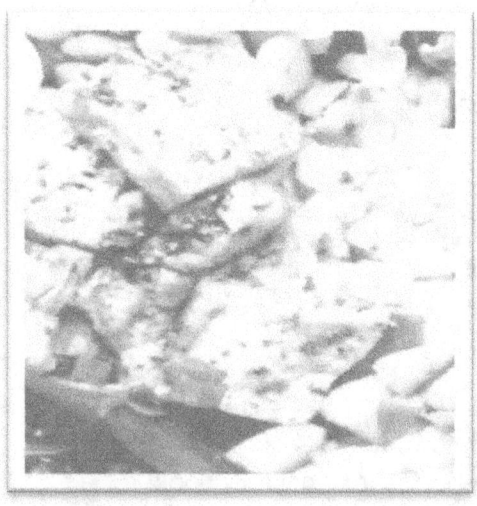

CHAPTER 4 DELICIOUS DINNER RECIPES

Chickpea and Quinoa Bowl: Add it up with Roasted Red Pepper Sauce:

Preparation Time:

- 30 minutes

Ingredients:

- 1 cup of cooked quinoa

- 1 can (15 oz) chickpeas, drained and rinsed

- 1 cup cherry tomatoes, halved

- 1 cucumber, diced

- 1/4 cup red onion, finely chopped

- 1/4 cup feta cheese, crumbled

- Use 1/4 cup of Kalamata olives, pitted and sliced.

- Fresh parsley for garnish

- Roasted Red Pepper Sauce (store-bought or homemade)

Instructions:

1. In a bowl, assemble cooked quinoa, chickpeas, cherry tomatoes, cucumber, red onion, feta cheese, and Kalamata olives.

2. Drizzle with roasted red pepper sauce.

3. Toss gently to combine.

4. Garnish with fresh parsley.

5. Serve and enjoy!

Nutritional Value Calories: 400

- Protein: 15g

- Fat: 15g

- Carbohydrates: 55g

- Fiber: 12g

Chickpea Tuna Salad:

Preparation Time:

- 15 minutes

Ingredients:

- 1 can (15 oz) chickpeas, drained and mashed

- 1 can (5 oz) tuna, drained

- 1/4 cup celery, finely chopped

- 1/4 cup red onion, finely chopped

- 2 tablespoons of mayonnaise

- 1 tablespoon Dijon mustard

- Salt and pepper to taste

- Lettuce leaves or bread for serving

Instructions:

1. In a bowl, combine mashed chickpeas, tuna, celery, red onion, mayonnaise, Dijon mustard, salt, and pepper.

2. Mix well.

3. Serve over lettuce leaves or as a sandwich filling.

4. Enjoy your Chickpea Tuna Salad!

Nutritional Value: Calories: 350

- Protein: 20g

- Fat: 15g

- Carbohydrates: 30g

- Fiber: 8g

Kale and Quinoa Salad with Lemon Dressing:

Preparation Time:

- 25 minutes

Ingredients:

- 2 cups of cooked quinoa

- Use 4 cups of kale, stems removed, and chopped

- 1 cup cherry tomatoes, halved

- 1/2 cup feta cheese, crumbled

- 1/4 cup red onion, thinly sliced

- 1/4 cup sunflower seeds

- Lemon Dressing: 2 tablespoons olive oil, 1 tablespoon lemon juice, salt, and pepper

Instructions:

1. In a large bowl, combine cooked quinoa, chopped kale, cherry tomatoes, feta cheese, red onion, and sunflower seeds.

2. You need to whisk together, in a small bowl, olive oil, lemon juice, salt, and pepper.

3. To combine, you have to pour the dressing over the salad and toss gently.

4. Serve and enjoy your nutritious Kale and Quinoa Salad!

Nutritional Value: Calories: 400

- Protein: 15g

- Fat: 20g

- Carbohydrates: 45g

- Fiber: 8g

Creamy Salmon Pasta with Sun-Dried Tomatoes:

Preparation Time:

- 20 minutes

Ingredients:

- 8 oz. pasta (of your choice)

- 1 tablespoon of olive oil

- 2 salmon fillets, cooked and flaked

- 1/2 cup sun-dried tomatoes, chopped

- 1/2 cup heavy cream

- 1/4 cup grated Parmesan cheese

- Fresh basil for garnish

- Salt and pepper to taste

Instructions:

1. Just try to cook the pasta following the package instructions.

2. In a pan, heat olive oil and sauté sun-dried tomatoes.

3. Add cooked and flaked salmon to the pan.

4. Pour in heavy cream and Parmesan cheese. Stir until creamy.

5. Season with salt and pepper.

6. Toss the cooked pasta into the creamy sauce.

7. Garnish with fresh basil.

8. Serve and enjoy your creamy salmon pasta!

Nutritional Value: Calories: 500

- Protein: 25g

- Fat: 25g

- Carbohydrates: 40g

- Fiber: 4g

White Bean and Sun-Dried Tomato Gnocchi:

Preparation Time:

- 25 minutes

Ingredients:

- 1 package (16 oz) potato gnocchi
- Use 1 can of (15 oz) white beans, drained and rinsed.
- 1/2 cup sun-dried tomatoes, chopped
- 2 tablespoons of olive oil
- 2 cloves garlic, minced
- 1/4 cup fresh basil, chopped
- Salt and pepper to taste
- Grated Parmesan cheese for serving

Instruction

1. You need to heat olive oil and sauté minced garlic in a pan.
2. Add white beans and sun-dried tomatoes to the pan.
3. Stir in cooked gnocchi.

4. Season with salt and pepper.

5. Garnish with fresh basil.

6. Serve with grated Parmesan cheese on top.

Nutritional Value: Calories: 450

- Protein: 15g

- Fat: 15g

- Carbohydrates: 65g

- Fiber: 8g

Quinoa Chili with Sweet Potatoes:

Preparation Time:

- 30 minutes

Ingredients:

- 1 cup quinoa, rinsed

- Use 1 can of (15 oz) black beans, drained and rinsed.

- Use 1 can of (15 oz.) kidney beans, drained and rinsed.

- 1 can (14 oz) diced tomatoes

- 1 cup sweet potatoes, diced

- 1 onion, chopped

- 2 cloves garlic, minced

- 1 tablespoon chili powder

- 1 teaspoon of cumin

- Salt and pepper to taste

- Vegetable broth (as needed)

Instructions:

1. In a large pot, sauté chopped onion and minced garlic.

2. Add diced sweet potatoes, black beans, kidney beans, and diced tomatoes to the pot.

3. Stir in quinoa, chili powder, cumin, salt, and pepper.

4. Pour in enough vegetable broth to cover the ingredients.

5. Simmer until the sweet potatoes and quinoa are cooked.

6. Adjust seasoning if needed.

7. Serve your hearty Quinoa Chili and enjoy!

Nutritional Value: Calories: 400

- Protein: 15g

- Fat

Top of Form

Skillet Lemon Chicken with Spinach

Preparation Time: 20 minutes
Ingredients:

- 4 boneless, skinless chicken breasts

- Salt and pepper to taste

- 2 tablespoons of olive oil

- 4 cloves garlic, minced

- 1 cup cherry tomatoes, halved

- 3 cups of fresh spinach

- Juice of 2 lemons

- Zest of 1 lemon

- 1/2 cup chicken broth

- Fresh parsley for garnish

Instructions:

1. You have to season the chicken breasts with salt and pepper.

2. Then you heat olive oil in a skillet over medium-high heat.

3. Cook the chicken until browned on both sides, about 5 minutes per side.

4. Add garlic, cherry tomatoes, and spinach. Cook until the spinach wilts.

5. Pour in the lemon juice, lemon zest, and chicken broth. Simmer for 5 minutes.

6. Garnish with fresh parsley before serving.

Nutritional Value: (per serving)

- Calories: 350

- Protein: 30g

- Carbohydrates: 8g

- Fat: 20g

- Fiber: 3g

Spinach and Artichoke Dip Pasta

Preparation Time: 25 minutes
Ingredients:

- 8 oz. of pasta of your choice

- Use 1 cup of frozen spinach, thawed and drained.

- 1 can artichoke hearts, chopped

- 1 cup of ricotta cheese

- 1 cup grated Parmesan cheese

- 2 cloves garlic, minced

- Salt and pepper to taste

- Red pepper flakes (optional)

Instructions:

1. Cook pasta according to package instructions.

2. In a bowl, mix spinach, artichoke hearts, ricotta, Parmesan, and garlic.

3. Drain the pasta and toss with the spinach-artichoke mixture.

4. Season with salt, pepper, and red pepper flakes, if desired.

Nutritional Value: (per serving)

- Calories: 450

- Protein: 18g

- Carbohydrates: 40g

- Fat: 24g

- Fiber: 5g

Salmon and Avocado Poke Bowl

Preparation Time: 15 minutes

Ingredients:

- 2 cups sushi rice, cooked

- 1 lb. fresh salmon, cubed

- 1 avocado, sliced

- 1 cucumber, julienned

- 1/4 cup soy sauce

- 1 tablespoon sesame oil

- 1 tablespoon of rice vinegar

- then garnish with sesame seeds and green onions.

Instructions:

1. Arrange rice in bowls and top with salmon, avocado, and cucumber.

2. In a small bowl, mix soy sauce, sesame oil, and rice vinegar. Drizzle it over the bowl.

3. You have to garnish with sesame seeds and green onions.

Nutritional Value: (per serving)

- Calories: 500

- Protein: 25g

- Carbohydrates: 60g

- Fat: 20g

- Fiber: 6g

White Bean and Veggie Salad

Preparation Time: 15 minutes
Ingredients:

- 2 cans of white beans, drained and rinsed

- 1 cup cherry tomatoes, halved

- 1 cucumber, diced

- 1/2 red onion, finely chopped

- 1/4 cup feta cheese, crumbled

- 2 tablespoons of olive oil

- 1 tablespoon balsamic vinegar

- Salt and pepper to taste

- Fresh basil for garnish

Instructions:

1. In a large bowl, combine white beans, cherry tomatoes, cucumber, red onion, and feta.

2. In a small bowl, you have to whisk together olive oil, balsamic vinegar, salt, and pepper.

3. To combine, you have to pour the dressing over the salad and toss.

4. Garnish with fresh basil before serving.

Nutritional Value: (per serving)

- Calories: 300

- Protein: 12g

- Carbohydrates: 40g

- Fat: 10g

- Fiber: 10g

Salmon Tacos with Pineapple Salsa

Preparation Time: 30 minutes
Ingredients:

- 1 lb. salmon fillets

- 8 small corn tortillas

- 1 cup of shredded cabbage

- 1 cup pineapple, diced

- 1/2 red onion, finely chopped

- 1 jalapeño, seeded and minced

- Juice of 1 lime

- 1/4 cup fresh cilantro, chopped

- Salt and pepper to taste

Instructions:

1. Season the salmon with salt and pepper and grill until cooked.

2. Warm tortillas and assemble tacos with salmon, shredded cabbage, and pineapple salsa.

3. For the salsa, mix pineapple, red onion, jalapeño, lime juice, cilantro, salt, and pepper.

Nutritional Value: (per serving)

- Calories: 400

- Protein: 20g

- Carbohydrates: 40g

- Fat: 18g

- Fiber: 6g

Vegan Coconut Chickpea Curry

Preparation Time: 40 minutes
Ingredients:

- 2 cans chickpeas, drained and rinsed

- 1 can of coconut milk

- 1 onion, finely chopped

- 3 cloves garlic, minced

- 1 tablespoon curry powder

- 1 teaspoon of turmeric

- 1 teaspoon of cumin

- 1 cup diced tomatoes

- 1 cup of spinach

- Salt and pepper to taste

- Fresh cilantro for garnish

Instructions:

1. In a large pot, you have to sauté the onion and garlic until softened.

2. Add chickpeas, coconut milk, curry powder, turmeric, and cumin. Simmer for 20 minutes.

3. Stir in diced tomatoes and spinach. Cook until the spinach wilts.

4. Season with salt and pepper. Garnish with fresh cilantro.

Nutritional Value: (per serving)

- Calories: 350

- Protein: 15g

- Carbohydrates: 45g

- Fat: 15g

- Fiber: 12g

Salmon-Stuffed Avocados:

Preparation Time: 15 minutes
Ingredients:

- 2 avocados, halved and pitted

- 1 cup cooked salmon, flaked

- 1/4 cup red onion, finely diced

- 2 tablespoons cilantro, chopped

- 1 tablespoon of lime juice

- Salt and pepper to taste

Instructions:

1. In a bowl, combine the flaked salmon, red onion, cilantro, and lime juice.

2. You have to season with salt and pepper to get a taste.

3. Spoon the salmon mixture into the halved avocados.

4. Serve immediately, and enjoy!

Nutritional Value: (per serving, approximate)

- Calories: 300

- Protein: 20g

- Fat: 22g

- Carbohydrates: 10g

- Fiber: 7g

Crispy Fish Taco Bowls:

Preparation Time: 30 minutes
Ingredients:

- 1 lb. white fish fillets

- 1 cup of cornmeal

- 1 teaspoon of cumin

- 1 teaspoon paprika

- Salt and pepper to taste

- 4 cups of cooked rice

- 1 cup black beans, drained and rinsed

- 1 cup cherry tomatoes, halved

- 1/2 cup red cabbage, shredded

- Lime wedges for serving

Instructions:

1. Preheat the oven to 400°F (200°C).

2. Combine cornmeal, cumin, paprika, salt, and pepper in a bowl.

3. Dredge the fish fillets in the cornmeal mixture and bake until crispy.

4. Assemble bowls with rice, black beans, cherry tomatoes, shredded cabbage, and crispy fish.

5. Serve with lime wedges and enjoy!

Nutritional Value: (per serving, approximate)

- Calories: 450

- Protein: 25g

- Fat: 8g

- Carbohydrates: 75g

- Fiber: 8g

Vegan Grain Bowl:

Preparation   Time: 20   minutes
Ingredients:

- 1 cup quinoa, cooked

- 1 cup roasted vegetables (e.g., broccoli, carrots, bell peppers)

- 1/2 cup hummus

- 1/4 cup pumpkin seeds

- Fresh parsley for garnish

- Olive oil for drizzling

Instructions:

1. Arrange cooked quinoa in bowls.

2. Top with roasted vegetables, hummus, and pumpkin seeds.

3. Garnish with fresh parsley, and drizzle with olive oil.

4. Mix well, and enjoy this wholesome vegan grain bowl!

CHAPTER 5

Mouthwatering Soup Recipes
Turkish Red Lentil Soup with Mint:

Preparation Time: 30 minutes
Ingredients:

- 1 cup red lentils, rinsed

- 1 large onion, finely chopped

- 2 carrots, chopped

- 2 potatoes, peeled and diced

- 3 cloves garlic, minced

- 1 tablespoon of tomato paste

- 1 teaspoon ground cumin

- 1 teaspoon paprika

- 6 cups of vegetable broth

- Salt and pepper to taste

- Fresh mint leaves for garnish

Instructions:

1. Sauté the onion and garlic in a large pot until they become soft.

2. Add carrots, potatoes, lentils, tomato paste, cumin, and paprika. Stir well.

3. You have to pour in the vegetable broth and boil it. Reduce heat, cover, and simmer until lentils and vegetables are tender.

4. Then you use an immersion blender and blend the soup until it becomes smooth.

5. Season with salt and pepper, and garnish with fresh mint leaves before serving.

Nutritional Value: *(values per serving)*

- Calories: 250

- Protein: 15g

- Fat: 1g

- Carbohydrates: 50g

- Fiber: 10g

Quinoa Vegetable Soup:

Preparation Time: 45 minutes
Ingredients:

- 1 cup quinoa, rinsed

- 1 onion, diced

- 2 carrots, sliced

- 2 celery stalks, chopped

- 1 zucchini, diced

- 1 can of diced tomatoes

- 6 cups of vegetable broth

- 1 teaspoon dried thyme

- 1 teaspoon dried oregano

- Salt and pepper to taste

- Fresh parsley for garnish

Instructions:

1. In a large pot, you have to sauté the onions until translucent. Add carrots, celery, and zucchini.

2. Stir in quinoa, diced tomatoes, vegetable broth, thyme, and oregano. Bring to a boil, and then simmer until the quinoa is cooked.

3. Season with salt and pepper, and garnish with fresh parsley before serving.

Nutritional Value: *(values per serving)*

- Calories: 280

- Protein: 12g

- Fat: 4g

- Carbohydrates: 50g

- Fiber: 8g

Roasted Red Bell Pepper Soup

Preparation Time: 50 minutes
Ingredients:

- Use 4 red bell peppers, roast them, and peel them.

- 1 onion, chopped

- 2 cloves garlic, minced

- 1 potato, peeled and diced

- 4 cups of vegetable broth

- 1 teaspoon smoked paprika

- Salt and pepper to taste

- Olive oil for roasting

- Fresh basil for garnish

Instructions:

1. Preheat the oven to 400°F (200°C). Roast the bell peppers until charred, then peel and chop them.

2. In a pot, sauté the onions and garlic until softened. Add diced potatoes, roasted bell peppers, and smoked paprika.

3. Pour in vegetable broth, bring to a boil, then simmer until potatoes are tender.

4. Blend the soup until it is smooth. Season with salt and pepper.

5. Garnish with a drizzle of olive oil and fresh basil before serving.

Nutritional Value: *(values per serving)*

- Calories: 180

- Protein: 3g

- Fat: 6g

- Carbohydrates: 30g

- Fiber: 5g

Curried Cauliflower Soup:

Preparation Time: 40 minutes
Ingredients:

- 1 large cauliflower, chopped

- 1 onion, diced

- 2 carrots, sliced

- 3 cloves garlic, minced

- 1 tablespoon curry powder

- 4 cups of vegetable broth

- 1 can of coconut milk

- Salt and pepper to taste

- Fresh cilantro for garnish

Instructions:

1. Sauté onions and garlic until translucent. Add cauliflower, carrots, and curry powder.

2. Pour in vegetable broth and coconut milk. Then bring it to a simmer and cook it until the vegetables are tender.

3. Blend the soup until it is creamy. Season with salt and pepper.

4. Garnish with fresh cilantro before serving.

Nutritional Value: *(values per serving)*

- Calories: 220

- Protein: 5g

- Fat: 15g

- Carbohydrates: 20g

- Fiber: 6g

Spicy Lime Avocado Soup:

Preparation Time: 20 minutes
Ingredients:

- 2 avocados, peeled and pitted

- 2 cups of vegetable broth

- Juice of 2 limes

- 1 jalapeño, seeded and chopped

- 1 clove garlic, minced

- Salt and pepper to taste

- Fresh cilantro for garnish

Instructions:

1. In a blender, combine avocados, vegetable broth, lime juice, jalapeño, and garlic. Blend until smooth.

2. Season with salt and pepper. Adjust the lime and spice levels to taste.

3. Garnish with fresh cilantro before serving.

Nutritional Value:

Calories: 180

- Protein: 3g

- Fat: 15g

- Carbohydrates: 10g

- Fiber: 6g

Dairy-Free Creamy Broccoli Soup:

Preparation Time: 35 minutes
Ingredients:

- 4 cups of broccoli florets

- 1 onion, chopped

- 2 cloves garlic, minced

- 1 potato, peeled and diced

- 4 cups of vegetable broth

- 1 cup of unsweetened almond milk

- 2 tablespoons of nutritional yeast

- Salt and pepper to taste

- Olive oil for sautéing

- Chopped chives for garnish

Instructions:

1. In a pot, sauté onions and garlic in olive oil until softened. Add diced potatoes and broccoli.

2. Pour in vegetable broth and simmer until vegetables are tender.

3. Then use a blender to puree the soup and allow it to be smoothed. Return to the pot.

4. Stir in almond milk and nutritional yeast. Season with salt and pepper.

5. Garnish with chopped chives before serving.

Nutritional Value: *(values per serving)*

- Calories: 150

- Protein: 5g

- Fat: 7g

- Carbohydrates: 20g

- Fiber: 5g

Sweet Potato and Kale Soup:

Preparation Time: 40 minutes
Ingredients:

- 2 sweet potatoes, peeled and diced

- 1 onion, chopped

- 2 carrots, sliced

- 3 cups kale, chopped

- 2 cloves garlic, minced

- 6 cups of vegetable broth

- 1 teaspoon ground cumin

- 1/2 teaspoon cinnamon

- Salt and pepper to taste

- Olive oil for sautéing

- Toasted pumpkin seeds for garnish

Instructions:

1. Sauté onions and garlic in olive oil until softened. Add sweet potatoes, carrots, and kale.

2. Pour in the vegetable broth and bring to a boil. Simmer until the sweet potatoes are tender.

3. Season with ground cumin, cinnamon, salt, and pepper.

4. Use an immersion blender to partially blend the soup for a chunky texture.

5. Garnish with toasted pumpkin seeds before serving.

Nutritional Value: Calories: 180

- Protein: 4g

- Fat: 3g

- Carbohydrates: 35g

- Fiber: 6g

Roasted Tomato Soup:

Preparation   Time: 50   minutes
Ingredients:

- 8 large tomatoes, halved

- 1 onion, sliced

- 3 cloves garlic, minced

- 2 carrots, sliced

- 4 cups of vegetable broth

- 2 tablespoons of olive oil

- 1 teaspoon dried thyme

- Salt and pepper to taste

- Fresh basil for garnish

Instructions:

1. Preheat the oven to 400°F (200°C). Place tomatoes, onions, garlic, and carrots on a baking sheet. Drizzle with olive oil and sprinkle with thyme, salt, and pepper. Roast until vegetables are caramelized.

2. Transfer roasted vegetables to a pot, add vegetable broth, and bring to a simmer. Cook until the carrots are tender.

3. Then, use a blender to puree the soup, allowing it to become smooth.

4. Season with additional salt and pepper, if needed.

5. Garnish with fresh basil before serving.

Nutritional Value: Calories: 160

- Protein: 4g

- Fat: 8g

- Carbohydrates: 20g

- Fiber: 5g

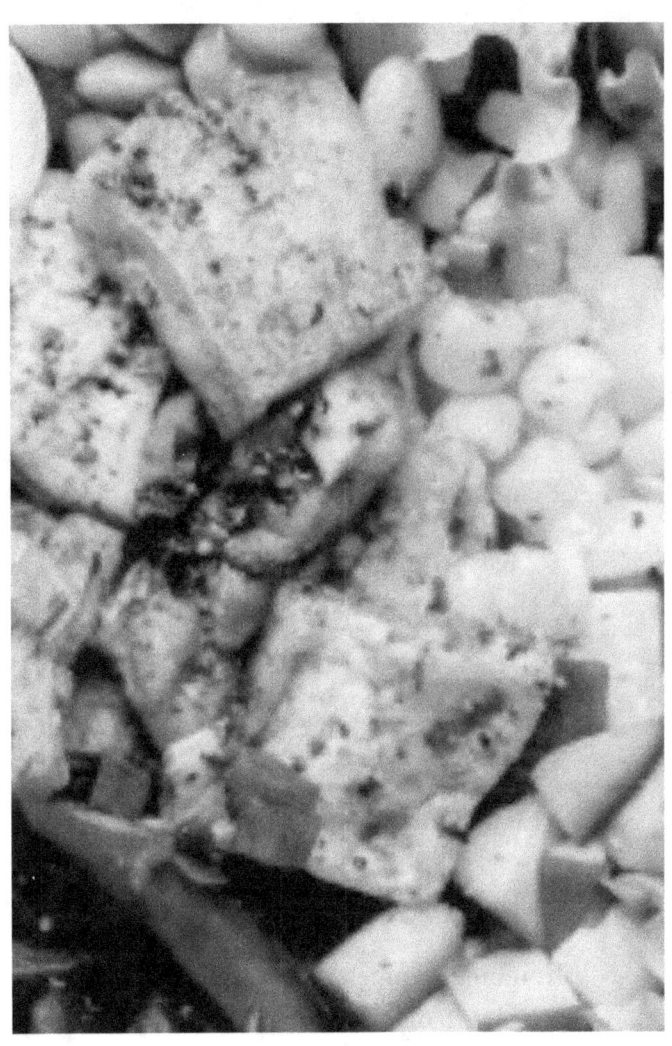

CHAPTER 6

Mouthwatering Smoothie Recipes
Pineapple-Turmeric Smoothie:

- Preparation Time:

- 5 minutes

- Ingredients:

- 1 cup of pineapple chunks

- 1/2 teaspoon turmeric powder

- 1/2 banana

- 1/2 cup Greek yogurt

- 1/2 cup of coconut water

- Ice cubes (optional)

- Instructions:

- Combine pineapple chunks, turmeric powder, banana, Greek yogurt, and coconut water in a blender.

- Blend until smooth.

- Add ice cubes if desired and blend again.

- Pour into a glass and enjoy!

- Nutritional Value:

- Calories:

- Protein:

- Fiber:

- Vitamin C:

- Potassium:

Kiwi and Kale Smoothie:

- Preparation Time:

- 7 minutes

- Ingredients:

- 2 kiwis, peeled and sliced

- 1 cup kale leaves, stems removed

- 1/2 green apple, cored and chopped

- 1/2 cucumber, peeled and sliced

- 1/2 lemon, juiced

- 1 cup of water

- Ice cubes (optional)

- Instructions:

- Place kiwis, kale, green apple, cucumber, and lemon juice in a blender.

- Add water and blend until smooth.

- Add ice cubes if desired and blend again.

- Pour into a glass and enjoy!

- Nutritional Value:

- Calories:

- Protein:

- Fiber:

- Vitamin K:

- Vitamin C:

Celery-Ginger Smoothie

- Preparation Time:

- 6 minutes

- Ingredients:

- 2 celery stalks, chopped

- 1/2 inch ginger, peeled and grated

- 1 green pear, cored and chopped

- 1/2 lemon, juiced

- 1/2 cup of coconut water

- Ice cubes (optional)

- Instructions:

- Combine celery, ginger, pear, lemon juice, and coconut water in a blender.

- Blend until smooth.

- Add ice cubes if desired and blend again.

- Pour into a glass and enjoy!

- Nutritional Value:

- Calories:

- Protein:

- Fiber:

- Potassium:

- Vitamin C:

Mango-Strawberries Smoothie

- Preparation Time:

- 5 minutes

- Ingredients:

- 1 cup of mango chunks

- 1/2 cup strawberries, hulled

- 1/2 banana

- 1/2 cup plain yogurt

- 1/2 cup almond milk

- Ice cubes (optional)

- Instructions:

- Combine mango chunks, strawberries, banana, yogurt, and almond milk in a blender.

- Blend until smooth.

- Add ice cubes if desired and blend again.

- Pour into a glass and enjoy!

- Nutritional Value:

- Calories:

- Protein:

- Fiber:

- Vitamin A:

- Vitamin C:

Grapefruit-Parsley Smoothie:

- Preparation Time:

- 6 minutes

- Ingredients:

- 1 grapefruit, peeled and segmented

- 1/2 cup of fresh parsley leaves

- 1/2 green apple, cored and chopped

- 1/2 cucumber, peeled and sliced

- 1/2 lime, juiced

- 1 cup of water

- Ice cubes (optional)

- Instructions:

- Place grapefruit segments, parsley, green apple, cucumber, and lime juice in a blender.

- Add water and blend until smooth.

- Add ice cubes if desired and blend again.

- Pour into a glass and enjoy!

- Nutritional Value:

- Calories:

- Protein:

- Fiber:

- Vitamin C:

- Folate:

Avocado Smoothie:

- Preparation Time:

- 5 minutes

- Ingredients:

- 1 ripe avocado, peeled and pitted

- 1/2 cup of spinach leaves

- 1/2 banana

- 1/2 cup Greek yogurt

- 1 tablespoon of honey

- 1 cup of almond milk

- Ice cubes (optional)

- Instructions:

- Combine avocado, spinach, banana, Greek yogurt, honey, and almond milk in a blender.

- Blend until smooth.

- Add ice cubes if desired and blend again.

- Pour into a glass and enjoy!

- Nutritional Value:

- Calories:

- Protein:

- Fiber:

- Healthy Fats:

- Vitamin K:

Berry Smoothie:

- Preparation Time:

- 4 minutes

- Ingredients:

- Use 1 cup of mixed berries (strawberries, blueberries, or raspberries).

- 1/2 banana

- 1/2 cup plain yogurt

- 1/2 cup of orange juice

- 1 tablespoon of chia seeds

- Ice cubes (optional)

- Instructions:

- Combine mixed berries, banana, yogurt, orange juice, and chia seeds in a blender.

- Blend until smooth.

- Add ice cubes if desired and blend again.

- Pour into a glass and enjoy!

- Nutritional Value:

- Calories:

- Protein:

- Fiber:

- Vitamin C:

- Antioxidants:

Carrot-Apple Smoothie

- Preparation Time:

- 6 minutes

- Ingredients:

- 1 carrot, peeled and chopped

- 1/2 apple, cored and chopped

- 1/2 cup plain yogurt

- 1 tablespoon flaxseeds

- 1/2 teaspoon cinnamon

- 1 cup of water

- Ice cubes (optional)

- Instructions:

- Combine carrot, apple, yogurt, flaxseeds, cinnamon, and water in a blender.

- Blend until smooth.

- Add ice cubes if desired and blend again.

- Pour into a glass and enjoy!

- Nutritional Value:

- Calories:

- Protein:

- Fiber:

- Vitamin A:

- Calcium:

Mango Raspberry Smoothie

- Preparation Time:

- 5 minutes

- Ingredients:

- 1 cup of mango chunks

- 1/2 cup raspberries

- 1/2 banana

- 1/2 cup coconut milk

- 1 tablespoon of hemp seeds

- Ice cubes (optional)

- Instructions:

- Combine mango chunks, raspberries, banana, coconut milk, and hemp seeds in a blender.

- Blend until smooth.

- Add ice cubes if desired and blend again.

- Pour into a glass and enjoy!

- Nutritional Value:

- Calories:

- Protein:

- Fiber:

- Healthy Fats:

- Vitamin C:

Avocado Green Smoothie

- Preparation Time:

- 7 minutes

- Ingredients:

- 1 ripe avocado, peeled and pitted

- 1 cup kale leaves, stems removed

- 1/2 green apple, cored and chopped

- 1/2 cucumber, peeled and sliced

- 1/2 lime, juiced

- 1 cup of water

- Ice cubes (optional)

- Instructions:

- Combine avocado, kale, green apple, cucumber, lime juice, and water in a blender.

- Blend until smooth.

- Add ice cubes if desired and blend again.

- Pour into a glass and enjoy!

- Nutritional Value:

- Calories:

- Protein:

- Fiber:

- Vitamin K:

- Vitamin C:

Mixed-Berry Breakfast Smoothie:

- Preparation Time:

- 6 minutes

- Ingredients:

- 1 cup mixed berries (strawberries, blueberries, blackberries)

- 1/2 cup oats

- 1/2 banana

- 1/2 cup Greek yogurt

- 1 tablespoon of honey

- 1 cup milk (dairy or plant-based)

- Ice cubes (optional)

- Instructions:

- Combine mixed berries, oats, bananas, Greek yogurt, honey, and milk in a blender.

- Blend until smooth.

- Add ice cubes if desired and blend again.

- Pour into a glass and enjoy!

- Nutritional Value:

- Calories:

- Protein:

- Fiber:

- Calcium:

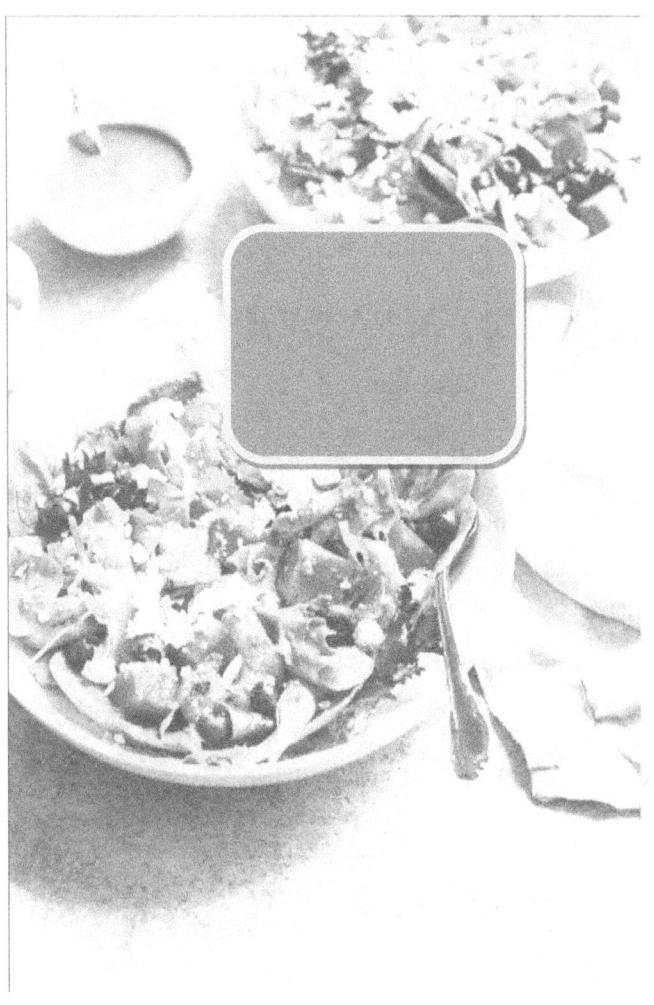

CHAPTER 7

Awesome Snacks and Desert

Lemon-Blueberry Poke Cake

Preparation Time:

- 15 minutes

Ingredients:

- 1 box lemon cake mix

- 1 cup blueberries

- 1 can sweetened condensed milk

- 1 cup lemon curd

- Whipped cream for topping

Instructions:

1. Prepare the lemon cake mix according to package instructions.

2. Once baked and cooled, use the end of a wooden spoon to poke holes into the cake.

3. Pour sweetened condensed milk over the cake, ensuring it fills the holes.

4. Spread lemon curd over the top of the cake.

5. Sprinkle blueberries over the cake.

6. Refrigerate for at least 2 hours before serving.

7. Top with whipped cream before serving.

Nutritional Value:

Calories: Approximately 300 per serving

- Protein: 3g

- Carbohydrates: 45g

- Fat: 12g

Strawberry-Chocolate Greek Yogurt Bark

Preparation Time:

- 10 minutes

Ingredients:

- 2 cups Greek yogurt

- 1 cup strawberries, sliced

- 1/2 cup dark chocolate, melted

Instructions:

1. You have to use parchment paper to line a baking sheet.

2. Spread Greek yogurt evenly on the sheet.

3. Add sliced strawberries on top.

4. Drizzle melted dark chocolate over the yogurt.

5. Freeze for at least 3 hours.

6. Break into pieces before serving.

Nutritional Value:

- Calories: Approximately 120 per serving
- Protein: 6g
- Carbohydrates: 15g
- Fat: 5g

Lemon-Blueberry Nice Cream

Preparation Time:

- 5 minutes

Ingredients:

- 2 frozen bananas

- 1 cup blueberries

- 1 tablespoon lemon juice

Instructions:

1. Blend frozen bananas, blueberries, and lemon juice until smooth.

2. Serve immediately.

Nutritional Value:

- Calories: Approximately 150 per serving

- Protein: 2g

- Carbohydrates: 38g

- Fat: 1g

Oatmeal Cookie Fruit Pizza

Preparation Time:

- 20 minutes

Ingredients:

- 1 cup rolled oats

- 1/2 cup almond butter

- 1/4 cup honey

- 1 teaspoon vanilla extract

- Mixed fruits for topping

Instructions:

1. Mix rolled oats, almond butter, honey, and vanilla extract.

2. Press the mixture onto a pizza pan to form a crust.

3. Bake at 350°F (175°C) for 10-12 minutes.

4. Allow the crust to cool before adding mixed fruits on top.

Nutritional Value:

- Calories: Approximately 200 per serving

- Protein: 5g

- Carbohydrates: 25g

- Fat: 10g

Apple Coffee Cake

Preparation Time:

- 25 minutes

Ingredients:

- 2 cups all-purpose flour

- 1 teaspoon baking powder

- 1/2 teaspoon baking soda

- 1/2 cup unsalted butter, softened

- 1 cup granulated sugar

- 2 large eggs

- 1 teaspoon vanilla extract

- 1 cup sour cream

- 2 cups peeled and diced apples

- Streusel topping (1/2 cup brown sugar, 1/4 cup all-purpose flour, 1/2 teaspoon cinnamon, 2 tablespoons melted butter)

Instructions:

1. Preheat oven to 350°F (175°C). Grease and flour a baking pan.

2. In a medium bowl, whisk together flour, baking powder, and baking soda.

3. In a large bowl, cream together butter and sugar until light and fluffy.

4. Beat in eggs one at a time, then stir in vanilla extract.

5. Gradually mix in the dry ingredients, alternating with sour cream.

6. Fold in diced apples.

7. Pour batter into the prepared pan.

8. In a small bowl, combine streusel topping ingredients and sprinkle over the batter.

9. Bake for 40-45 minutes or until a toothpick inserted into the center comes out clean.

Nutritional Value:

- Calories: Approximately 300 per serving

- Protein: 4g

- Carbohydrates: 40g

- Fat: 14g

Chocolate Rye Babka

Preparation Time: 3 hours (including rising time)

Ingredients:

- 1 cup warm milk

- 2 1/4 teaspoons active dry yeast

- 1/2 cup granulated sugar

- 4 cups rye flour

- 1/2 teaspoon salt

- 1/2 cup unsalted butter, softened

- 2 large eggs

- 1 teaspoon vanilla extract

- 1/2 cup chocolate chips

- 1/4 cup cocoa powder

- 1/2 cup powdered sugar (for dusting)

Instructions:

1. In a bowl, combine warm milk, yeast, and a pinch of sugar. Allow it to settle for 5-10 minutes until foamy.

2. In a large mixing bowl, combine rye flour, sugar, and salt. Add the yeast mixture, softened butter, eggs, and vanilla extract. Mix until a dough forms.

3. Knead the dough on a floured surface until smooth. Place it in a greased bowl, cover, and let it rise for 1-2 hours.

4. Roll out the dough into a rectangle. Spread melted chocolate over the surface and sprinkle with cocoa powder.

5. Roll the dough tightly into a log, then cut it in half lengthwise. Twist the two halves together and place in a greased loaf pan.

6. Let it rise for another hour. Bake it at 350°F (175°C) allow it for 30-35 minutes.

7. Once cooled, dust with powdered sugar before serving.

Nutritional Value:

- Serving Size: 1 slice

- Calories: 220

- Protein: 5g

- Fat: 10g

- Carbohydrates: 30g

- Fiber: 3g

Chocolate Nut Bark

Preparation Time: 15 minutes

Ingredients:

- 8 ounces dark chocolate, chopped

- use 1 cup of mixed nuts (almonds, walnuts, pistachios), chopped

- 1/4 cup dried fruits (cranberries, apricots), chopped

- Sea salt for sprinkling

Instructions:

1. Melt the dark chocolate using a double boiler or in the microwave in 30-second intervals.

2. Line a baking sheet with parchment paper. Spread the melted chocolate evenly.

3. Sprinkle chopped nuts and dried fruits over the chocolate.

4. Allow it to set in the refrigerator for at least 1 hour.

5. Once set, break into pieces and sprinkle with sea salt.

Nutritional Value:

- Serving Size: 1 ounce

- Calories: 150

- Protein: 3g

- Fat: 10g

- Carbohydrates: 15g

- Fiber: 2g

3. Nuts and Nut Butters with Whole-Grain Crackers:

Preparation Time: 5 minutes

Ingredients:

- Assorted nuts (almonds, cashews, pecans)
- Nut butters (peanut butter, almond butter)
- Whole-grain crackers

Instructions:

1. Arrange a variety of nuts on a serving platter.
2. Place different nut butters in small bowls.
3. Serve with whole-grain crackers for dipping.

Nutritional Value:

- Serving Size: 1 ounce nuts + 2 tablespoons nut butter + 5 crackers
- Calories: 250
- Protein: 8g

- Fat: 18g

- Carbohydrates: 18g

- Fiber: 4g

Fish on Whole-Grain Crackers

Preparation Time: 10 minutes

Ingredients:

- Canned tuna or salmon

- Whole-grain crackers

- Lemon wedges

- Fresh dill for garnish

Instructions:

1. Drain the canned fish and flake it with a fork.

2. Place spoonfuls of fish on whole-grain crackers.

3. Garnish with fresh dill and serve with lemon wedges.

Nutritional Value:

- Serving Size: 5 crackers with fish

- Calories: 180

- Protein: 15g

- Fat: 8g

- Carbohydrates: 15g

- Fiber: 3g

Berry Chia Seed Pudding

Preparation Time: 4 hours (including chilling time)

Ingredients:

- use 1 cup of mixed berries (strawberries, blueberries, raspberries)

- 1/4 cup chia seeds

- 1 cup almond milk

- 1 tablespoon honey or maple syrup

- 1 teaspoon vanilla extract

Instructions:

1. Blend berries until smooth. Mix in chia seeds, almond milk, honey, and vanilla extract.

2. Refrigerate for at least 3-4 hours or overnight, stirring occasionally.

3. Serve chilled, topped with additional berries if desired.

Nutritional Value:

- Serving Size: 1 cup

- Calories: 120

- Protein: 4g

- Fat: 6g

- Carbohydrates: 15g

- Fiber: 8g

Veggies and Bean Dip

Preparation Time: 15 minutes

Ingredients:

- Assorted raw veggies (carrots, bell peppers, cucumber)

- use 1 can of black beans, drain it and rinse it

- 2 cloves garlic, minced

- Juice of 1 lime

- 2 tablespoons olive oil

- Salt and pepper to tasteInstructions:

1. Arrange sliced veggies on a platter.

2. In a food processor, blend black beans, garlic, lime juice, and olive oil until smooth.

3. Season with salt and pepper.

4. Serve the dip with the veggies.

Nutritional Value:

- Serving Size: 1/2 cup dip + assorted veggies

- Calories: 150

- Protein: 6g

- Fat: 7g

- Carbohydrates: 18g

- Fiber: 6g

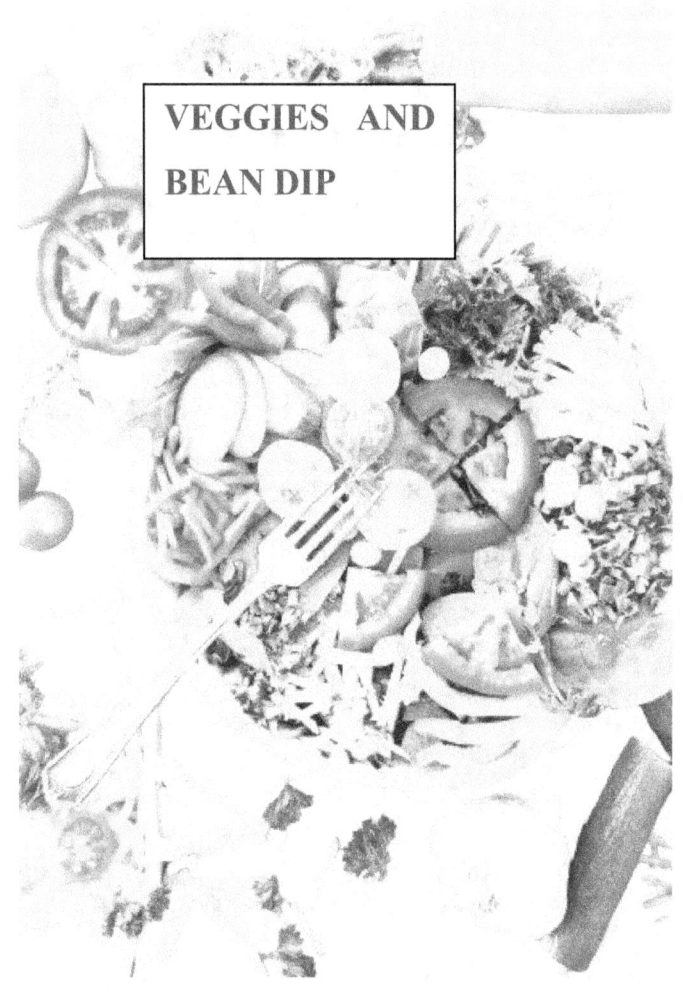

VEGGIES AND BEAN DIP

CHAPTER 8

8-week meal plan

Week 1

Day 1:

- Breakfast: Oatmeal with berries and walnuts

- Lunch: You will eat grilled salmon; add it quinoa and steamed broccoli.

- Snack: Greek yogurt with sliced strawberries

- Dinner: Stir-fried tofu with vegetables and brown rice

Day 2:

- Breakfast: Whole grain toast with avocado and poached eggs

- Lunch: Lentil soup with a side salad (spinach, cherry tomatoes, cucumber)

- Snack: mixed nuts (almonds, walnuts, and pistachios)

- Dinner: Baked chicken breast with sweet potato and green beans

Day 3:

- Breakfast: Smoothie with spinach, banana, and blueberries

- Lunch: eat quinoa salad and add chickpeas, cherry tomatoes, and feta cheese.

- Snack: You will eat hummus; add carrot and cucumber sticks.

- Dinner: You will eat grilled shrimp; add quinoa and roasted Brussels sprouts.

Day 4:

- Breakfast: just garnish Greek yogurt parfait, add granola, and mix berries.

- Lunch: Turkey and avocado wrap with whole grain tortilla

- Snack: sliced apple with almond butter

- Dinner: Baked cod with brown rice and asparagus

Day 5:

- Breakfast: Chia seed pudding with mango and kiwi

- Lunch: You will eat vegetable stir-fry; add it tofu and brown rice.

- Snack: Cottage cheese with pineapple chunks

- Dinner: Quinoa-stuffed bell peppers with ground turkey

Week 2

Day 6:

- Breakfast: You will eat whole-grain pancakes and add fresh berries.

- Lunch: Chicken and vegetable skewers with quinoa

- Snack: Trail mix with dried fruits and seeds

- Dinner: spaghetti squash with tomato sauce and lean ground beef

Day 7:

- Breakfast: scrambled eggs with spinach and whole grain toast

- Lunch: lentil and vegetable curry with basmati rice

- Snack: Celery sticks with peanut butter

- Dinner: Grilled swordfish with sweet potato wedges and green peas

Day 8:

- Breakfast: Smoothie with kale, pineapple, and banana

- Lunch: It will be a quinoa bowl. Eat it with black beans, corn, avocado, and salsa.

- Snack: Berries and cottage cheese

- Dinner: Baked chicken thighs with roasted vegetables and quinoa

Day 9:

- Breakfast: You will eat overnight oats; add almond milk, chia seeds, and mixed berries.

- Lunch: Turkey and vegetable stir-fry with brown rice

- Snack: yogurt with sliced peaches

- Dinner: Salmon with steamed broccoli and quinoa

Day 10:

- Breakfast: Whole grain toast with smoked salmon and cream cheese

- Lunch: chickpea salad with cucumbers, tomatoes, and feta cheese

- Snack: mixed nuts (almonds, walnuts, cashews)

- Dinner: You will eat baked cod. Eat it with quinoa and sautéed spinach.

Weeks 3&4

Repeat week 1 and 2.

Week 5:

Day 1:

- Breakfast: Smoothie with kale, pineapple, and ginger

- Lunch: Quinoa salad with cherry tomatoes, cucumber, and grilled chicken

- Snack: You will eat Greek yogurt. Eat it with honey and sliced almonds.

- Dinner: Baked salmon with sweet potato wedges and asparagus

Day 2:

- Breakfast: Chia seed pudding with mixed berries

- Lunch: It will be lentil and vegetable soup with a side of whole-grain bread.

- Snack: apple slices with almond butter

- Dinner: stir-fried tofu with broccoli and brown rice

Day 3:

- Breakfast: Oatmeal with sliced banana and walnuts

- Lunch: Turkey and avocado wrap with whole grain tortilla

- Snack: Cottage cheese with pineapple chunks

- Dinner: You will eat. Grilled shrimp, quinoa, and roasted Brussels sprouts

Day 4:

- Breakfast: Your breakfast should be Whole-grain pancakes Eat it with fresh berries.

- Lunch: This should be chickpea and spinach curry; add brown rice.

- Snack: mixed nuts (almonds, walnuts, and pistachios)

- Dinner: Baked cod with quinoa and sautéed kale

Day 5:

- Breakfast: You will eat a Greek yogurt parfait; add granola and mixed berries.

- Lunch: Quinoa-stuffed bell peppers with lean ground beef

- Snack: Eat hummus and add carrot and cucumber sticks.

- Dinner: spaghetti squash with tomato sauce and grilled chicken

Week 6

Day 6:

- Breakfast: Whole grain toast with avocado and poached eggs

- Lunch: Grilled chicken Caesar salad with plenty of leafy greens

- Snack: Trail mix with dried fruits and seeds

- Dinner: Baked turkey meatballs with quinoa and roasted vegetables

Day 7:

- Breakfast: this will be scrambled eggs; add spinach and whole grain toast.

- Lunch: This will be lentil and vegetable stir-fry; add tofu and brown rice.

- Snack: this will be berries and cottage cheese.

- Dinner: This will be baked salmon. Eat it with quinoa and steamed broccoli.

Day 8:

- Breakfast: This will be Overnight oats are eaten with almond milk, chia seeds, and mixed berries.

- Lunch: this will be turkey and vegetable kebabs; also add a side of couscous.

- Snack: This will be a sliced apple with almond butter.

- Dinner: eat Grilled swordfish is eaten with sweet potato wedges and green peas.

Day 9:

- Breakfast: Smoothie with spinach, banana, and blueberries

- Lunch: This will be a quinoa bowl. Eat it with black beans, corn, avocado, and salsa.

- Snack: You will eat yogurt with sliced peaches.

- Dinner: stir-fried shrimp with vegetables and brown rice

Day 10:

- Breakfast: Whole grain toast with smoked salmon and cream cheese

- Lunch: Mediterranean-style lentil salad with feta cheese and olives

- Snack: Celery sticks with peanut butter

- Dinner: Baked chicken thighs with quinoa and sautéed spinach

Week 7&8

Repeat week 5 and 6.

Daily Meal Planner

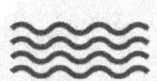

WEEK:　　　　**MONTH:**

BREAKFAST	LUNCH

DINNER	SNACKS

NOTES

Daily Meal Planner

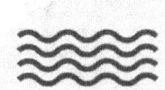

WEEK :   **MONTH :**

BREAKFAST	LUNCH

DINNER	SNACKS

NOTES

Daily Meal Planner

WEEK :   MONTH :

BREAKFAST	LUNCH

DINNER	SNACKS

NOTES

Daily Meal Planner

WEEK :   MONTH :

BREAKFAST

LUNCH

DINNER

SNACKS

NOTES

Daily Meal Planner

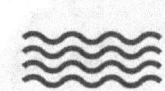

WEEK: **MONTH:**

BREAKFAST	LUNCH

DINNER	SNACKS

NOTES

www.ingramcontent.com/pod-product-compliance
Lightning Source LLC
Chambersburg PA
CBHW071046290526
45795CB00004B/1352